Rebuilding the Mind

Poetry by Gavin Jackson

Rebuilding the Mind

A Journey of Recovery Through Poetry

By Gavin Jackson

Gavin Jackson worked as a Managing Director for a top Global Bank based in London. He had everything he wanted in life, The Family, the home, the career...until one day everything went black.

Rushing home from work one day to be with his ailing father, he suffered a heart attack on the steps of Liverpool Street Station. A British Transport Police Officer witnessed the incident and was on the scene instantly performing CPR. This person is one of many who saved Gavin's life that day.

He was rushed to Saint Bartholomews Hospital in London where his family waited anxiously for news. They were told that he had suffered a serious cardiac event and that he had been 'down' for 55 minutes before paramedics were able to start his heart again.

The Doctors had put him in an artificial coma as they monitored his condition, but the family were told to be prepared for the worst, that he may not wake up at all and that if he did, it was unlikely that he would progress beyond a vegetative state.

The family waited day in day out for news, meanwhile Gavin fought for his life. Some days there was no news, other days set backs, but gradually, day by day, tiny miracles would occur. He began to breathe on his own. He began to make sounds and finally, he opened his eyes. He began to recognise his family and remeber little things, names, people, memories. Doctors were baffled at his recovery and he is, to this day , used as an exceptional case study in medicine. He had less than a 3% chance of regaining consciousness after the extent of his oxygen deprivation.

Several weeks later,He was moved to a rehabilitation facility to strengthen his body and mind. After months of hard work and dedication from both Gavin and his Wife, he came home. Now, he is a different man. He is able to go about his day to day life living with his wife and regularly visits his family. He volunteers for the UK wide charity 'Headway' which provides support not only to victims of brain injury, but also to their families.

It was shortly after his road to recovery that he began writing poetry. He had never been a poet before his incident. But now, he regularly wakes up in the middle of the night with ideas and is inspired to write, both about his experiences in life, but also his observations and feelings of the world around him.

This book is dedicated to all of the Doctors, Paramedics, British Transport Police Officers, family, nurses and friends who have been by Gavins side throughout this journey.Here is a book which shares an insight into the way Gavin has used poetry to express his own experiences and heal from the inside out.

All Proceeds will be donated to Headway SELNWK

It Happened On a Tuesday

It happened on a Tuesday running for a train

It was a November morning pouring down with rain.

Then I just collapsed proper hit the deck not able to
breath or speak

It was like a train wreck, medics on me straight away
doing CPR .

With hard work kept me going, for the next hour.

Ambulance to the hospital, they took me to Saint
Barts

Speeding through the traffic to try to fix my heart.

Straight into intensive care,tubes in every hole,

They worked in me for hours, to fix me me was their
goal.

Was put into a coma,and transferred to a side ward,

They kept me heavily sedated, hoping for some
reward.

When I first opened my eyes,tears came on that day

Recognition came soon after,although my eyes were grey.

First face I saw was Lorraines, who hadn't left me alone.

4 months in the Wellington,before I could go home.

Now I have been home,for 6 months to the dot,

I'm Feeling so much better, with help I've progressed a lot.

So what lies in the future ?I think about it all night

with help, from family and friends alike,my future is now very bright.

I now must say, that the person, who helps me see an end

is Lorraine, my lover, my soulmate, the one I call 'best friend'

Dazed and Confused.

Dazed and confused.
I've lost my way, I'm a long way from home.
I'm lost in a foreign land, I'm a long way from home.
I ask around but no one knows, I'm a foreigner and a long way from home.
I ask for help but no one understands me, I speak in a foreign tongue, I'm a long way from home.
I'm dazed and confused, I'm lost and a long way from home.

Lying on a beach

Lying on a beach with you

Is all I want to do

I want to wake in the morning

When the day is dawning

And to know that you are here,

beside me for the whole year

I'm such a lucky guy

even though I make you cry

I love you

and you love me too

together forever is what people say

So lying on a beach every day

is where we're most happy in every way

so why don't you join us down at the beach ?

so we can all learn, we can all teach.

Warrior

The war is done, the battle won,
The warrior can go home.
... but what lies beyond?

What does the future hold ? The warrior feels alone.
Back to his house, the place he felt safe, the place that
he called home.
Empty house, his family gone, the warrior feels alone.
His wife departed and took the kids,The warrior feels
alone.
Back in the house, the family house but it's no longer his
home
So what can he do, he can't stay there, he can not be
alone,
So the warrior leaves, goes back do war, so he won't be
alone.
Back with his comrades, back with his pals,
the warrior is now back home.

The Long Walk

I walk a long dark road,
Mile after mile, hour after hour.
I turn around and there's nothing there, no light, no one
there.
So I walk on, mile after mile, hour after hour.
I feels like I've been away for ages.

I had to go, I let them down, they relied on me, but
where was I in my head ?
So I walk on, mile after mile, hour after hour until ahead I
see a small light, which grows larger as I walk.
Then I can see now. There they are, all there, they were
there for me all along.

The long walk is over.

Sunshine State

Sunshine state of mind
As soon as we touch down, and I feel my feet on the
ground. I know I'm in a sunshine state of mind.
The brightness of the sun doesn't hurt my eyes, the wet
heat comes as no surprise, boy I know I'm in a
sunshine state of mind.
The temperature rises along with my mood, the grin on
my face could seem to some quite rude.
But I just don't care, coz
I'm in a sunshine state of mind.
Catching up with old friends and making some new, is
why we are here, it's what we wanna do. I'm totally in a
sunshine state of mind.
The hot Florida sun, so warm on my skin is like an old
friend welcoming us in.
So much to see here, and so much to do. We're so spoilt
for choice, the parks or the pool.
The pool wins the game, well just for today, we'll be out
there tomorrow, we'll go out to play, coz we're in a
sunshine state of mind.
And when summer is done and it's time to go home, and
the short dark days and long cold nights are chilling our
bones we won't care, we'll have our memories to keep us
warm.
Because we'll be forever be in a
sunshine state of mind.

The Big Man

William. I have lost so many memories of you
but I do remember that you were my friend,
one of my mentors
and you taught me a lot.
About life , about love, about friendship.
You were always there with a laugh and a stupid joke,
when all others were sad.
Always there to build and repair
and lend us the tools (that we often 'forgot' to return) to
do the job.
I remember the pool marathons down at the Nap and all
of the arguments it caused,
with you winding them all up.
I remember the time you showed the kids the spoon fish
in Florida and went into the sea when there were sharks
in the sea.
When it turned out it was only a Manatee and freaking
Rose out hahahaha.
I remember the Sunday lunches and your inventive way
of cooking !
What upsets me that I was not again there for you when
you passed.
There is a lot I don't remember,
but I do know that we love you, think about you and
miss you every day.
To me you've been a second Dad, confidant, councillor
and friend.

Seasons

Spring is here it's about new life,
new beginnings.
It brings new hopes, new dreams to dream.
Summer doesn't come soon enough.

Much needed sunshine, and the hot summer days, and
the long summer nights. School is out, it's time play.

Autumn brings it's own colours, orange, red and brown
in the falling leaves. It brings with it beautiful sunsets,
but with nights drawing in.
Playtime is over, schools are back in.
Its time to get your coats out of the closet, because.......

WINTER IS COMING.
And now winter is here, short cold days and colder long
nights.
First up the miserable November rains but soon enough
it's December and the snow is falling, covering all in its
blanket of comfort.
It's time to sleep, a time to regenerate, then spring will
come around again soon bringing new life, new
beginnings, new hopes and new dreams.

The Showman

Showman takes the stage.
Band pumps up and off we go.
Show starts with a bang, get in to the flow.
Stereos will whip 'em up, into some Robbie with his Rock
DJ to keep the tempo up.
Next you know it's Thriller, the Jacksons (sic) in control.
Time to slow it down
so bring on Bromley Ed,
everyone loves the Ed.
Bring it back up, with a classic crowd pleaser,
it's the Disney medley ·
WHAT ???
Oh yeah baby,
he's got'em hooked.
Finale is a massive mosh-up rap battle
(we're runnin' runnin' runnin', runnin' runnin' runnin')
That leaves 'em hangin'
and screaming for more, but there is no more, thats it for
now,
you've had your fill.
Showman leaves the stage,
he'll be back soon, he's hooked as much as you are.

Wide Awake

It's 2am she's wide awake, her mind is full of thoughts
Worried about the present,worried about the past
Worried about the future.
It's 3am she's wide awake.
Cleaning out the closets
Throwing away the past
God, what I thinking about back then when I bought
that?
It's 4am and still no sleep staring at the clock
Wondering where he is now and if he's coming back.

But she remembers that he is gone forever went off on a
mission and never came back.
It's 5am so she gets out of bed and goes downstairs to
feed the cat
who is still around , always there, her only real friend .
It's 6am and time to shower, get dressed and head off
out to work.
Where she'll smile and say 'hi' and pretend that it's ok .
She's not ok, she's hurting for the love she lost.
But life goes on and she shrugs to herself, I now must
just get on.

Lonely

As you walk about, day after day,
You'll see me sitting there cross legged on the floor.
Yes I'm looking for a kind of handout but do you know
what it's for ?
No it's not for booze or drugs.
It's not even for food , I just want to talk, I don't mean to
be rude.
I'm lonely and need to find some friends, because all the
others have good homes, their families, it's my fault I
suppose in the end,
I could have gone with them , but oh no, I knew best I
thought I'd be alright ,and make new friends but no,
there's no one.
No one stops to say hello, just to give a little time.
So do me a favour if you see me on the street please
don't just nod.
Say hello, I just want to talk, to make a new friend. It
might just benefit us both in the end.

Colours

It's not the colour of your *skin*, it's not the colour of your *eyes* , it's not the colour of you *hair*, what matters is the colour of your *heart*.
White is the colour of a snow capped mountain, when you're feeling on top of the world.
Yellow is the colour of summer, sunny days when you're warm, happy and relaxed in that warm summer sun.
Green is the colour of envy, when you're feeling that life is passing you by.
Red is the colour of anger, which for whatever reason makes you want to do harm.
Black is the colour of night, of darkness and the end of time.
It's not the colour of your skin, it's not the colour of your eyes , it's not the colour of you hair, what matters is the colour of your heart.

Beautiful People

North vs South,East vs West,

Rich vs Poor No Winners, all Losers
Just caught in the crossfire
Such beautiful people
Such a beautiful place
But why did this happen ?
But how did this happen ?
Pure greed, Pure jealousy
Pure avarice, Pure wickedness
So many children
So many innocents
So many tears
And then you just left
You left the children
You left the innocents
No place for them
No food for them,
No shelter for them
No schools for them
No hospitals for them
Yet they survived
Such courage, such bravery
And now they have
Rebuilt their homes.
Rebuilt their schools
Rebuilt their hospitals
and now can look to the future.
The beautiful and courageous people of Vietnam.

Reverse Gear

We talk and talk ... and talk again.

About the same old stuff, over and over again.
You tell me the truth but I think it's not true.
So you tell me again, so why don't I believe you ?

I tell you you're wrong, that you don't understand.
But you're just trying to help, I know there's a plan.
But to fix this brain, is not easy to do.
Just call up the 'shop'? book me in for a quick over-do ?

It's not easy as that, I wish it were true.
No, this truck is properly broke, the engine just blew.
And now I'm stuck in reverse gear, there's nothing I can
do.

Altered State

I'm in an altered state.
As a young man I dreamed a lot about the future.
I had it all.
My wife my kids my work my dreams.
I had it all planned out, I had it all.
As I grew up to be a man, I still had that same future.
My career, the travel, the holidays with family and
friends, the future looked safe and rosey.
I had it all.
Dreams can come true ?
Then it changed one November morning.
I'm in an altered state.
I still have those dreams but they have changed.
My hopes and plans have all changed.
Have they gone ?
No !
They've only changed.
No more 5am starts, no more midnight ends.
I've left all that behind.
Looking to the future, to make some new dreams.
I'm in an altered state.

Empty Vessels

Empty vessels in an empty house.
You were elected to serve
So even when you actually attend, what purpose do you
serve ?
Who do you serve ?
Is it the homeless guy ? Who fought for our freedom ?
Or the single mother of three, who
can't feed or clothe her kids
Who do you serve ?
Is it the struggling small business who can't pay their
staff ?
Who do you serve ?
Or is it your friends at the silver spoon club ? who give
you back handers to secure their loyalty
Or by opening church fetes (?) or hosting rotary club
lunches with your friend the lord mayor ?
Please tell me just who do you serve
and how do you serve us ?

Friends

Friends can be new or old.
Friends can be young or old.
Friends will welcome you.
Friends won't leave you out in the cold.
Friends can be girls or boys, they can love you equally.
Friends will not judge by whether you're fat or thin, or
the colour of your skin.
Friends know when to speak up or when to shut the fuck
up.
Friends will tell you if your hair is a mess, or you're too
big for that dress.
Friends will be with you forever, near or far they'll be in
your heart and mind.
Thank you all, for being my friend,
you'll never know how much it means to me.

The Lonely Old Man

The lonely old man sits in his chair, alone with his
thoughts, he's going nowhere.
He's no one to talk to and nobody cares, so the lonely
old man just sits in his chair.
He looks out the window and what does he see ?
It's only his reflection.
No one sees me.
So he sits in his chair day after day,
this ruffled old man, whose hair and eyes turning grey.
The lonely old man died in that chair, with no one to talk
to and no one to care.

My World

You are my world, there's no other to say it.
You are my world, don't you ever forget it.
You are my world, don't ever change it.
You are my world, you're always there for me.
You are my world, you make me happy, as happy as I
could ever be.
You are my world, I'd be lost without you.
You are my world, and I know your love is true.
So let's grow old together, and make our dreams come
true.
Merry Christmas darling (wherever you are hahahaha).
All my love.

Sometimes

Sometimes I can be happy without having to smile.
Sometimes I can be sad but not shed a tear.
Sometimes I can be loud but not always shout.
Sometimes I can be quiet and don't need to talk.
Sometimes I'm angry and don't understand, try as I
might, it just makes no sense to me.
Sometimes I'm confused and can't find my way.
So please forgive me, I'm not being rude, but sometimes
I just don't understand.

The Angry Man

The angry man lives within us all,
sometimes he's big and other times small.
He is always with you, he'll never go away.
He lives in your mind, all night and every day.
He's lost all his family, he's lost all his friends, but he says
he is happy "just leave me alone".
If you ever talk to him, ask him "what's the problem ?"
the angry man just frowns and replies "go away just
leave me alone"

Maroon and Gold

On Saturdays, in autumn though to spring.
You'll found me down in Bexley, to watch Rugby, drink
and sing.
Although my playing days are done now, I've still got the
bug.
So come on down to old Dartfordians, Kent's finest
rugby club.

The Crash

Blinding white light, then CRASH, it all goes black.
Oh crap I've had a heart attack.
Black for the longest time, then gradual shades of grey.
Hoping that the "weather" will improve, day by day by day.
But now the golden sun is coming out, just a little at a time.
So now this poem is done, I hope you liked my rhyme.

I Miss You Dad

I miss you Dad.
It's been hard to say until now.
I miss you Dad.
But now I'm coming to terms with it.
Remember the days we spent me annoying you in the
shed.
Remember the bird shows we went to when you'd get all
the prizes, I was so proud of you.
Remember the track days at brands hatch to watch the
bikes or the cars.
Remember me asking you if I could get a bike only to be
turned down every time.
I remember the times you would come out to help me
fix my car after finding me hitting it with a hammer, no
matter how busy you were.
I remember the times you would come up to my place to
help build my back deck. It's still standing well , thanks
to you.
Remember the times I needed a certain tool , no matter
what ever it was and you'd find one in the shed.
Remember the days and evenings we spent watching the
Grand Prix, while eating Mum's treacle pud !
What upsets me is not remembering your final days,
sitting by you side every evening.
What upsets me is that I was not at your side the day
you passed away.
I miss you Dad x

Innocents and Innocence

Let's talk about teenage knife crime
Why does this happen ?
Who is to blame ?
None of this makes any sense
Why did YOU do that ?
What did they do to YOU ?
Did they look at YOU the wrong way ?
Why did YOU do that ?
Was it the colour of their skin ?
Was it their religion ?
Why did YOU do that ?
Or maybe the colour of their shirt ?
How did this happen ?
Why did YOU do that ?
They were killed while serving OUR country
They were killed for being young. They were killed while
protecting the public
They were killed while protecting their family
All of them were innocent.
So please please tell me,
WHY did YOU do that ?

Acknowledgments

I owe so many thanks to so many people that I cannot mention you all by name (you know who you are). I will always be grateful for everything you have done for me .

I do however, want to mention;

First and foremost my lovely wife Lorraine, without whose love and support I would not be here today.

My children, Mike, Liam, Chloe, their partners and my wonderful grandchildren.

My amazing mum who lost her husband on the day of my heart attack and who has been a source of strength for us despite her hardship.

Mariano for your guidance and continued support.

Rebecca who has been with us since day one of this journey, both physically and figuratively.

The Britsh Transport Police and London Ambulance Service who were first on the scene and who unquestionably saved my life.

All the staff at St Barts and The Wellington Hospitals who kept me alive and brought me back to health.

Cover Photography by Lorraine Jackson

Poetry by Gavin Jackson

One mans Journey from near death back to life told through poetry.

Gavin Jackson is a Managing Director who has worked in the city for over 40 years. During a journey home from work, he suffered a near fatal heart attack. After weeks in a coma and months of rehab, Gavin emerged with a newfound talent. Poetry has become his means of expressing his own experiences, from losing loved ones, to his views on the world today.